Diet

by Lulu Hunt Peters

Chicago The Reilly and Lee Co.

1918

Dedicated by permission to

Herbert Hoover

Read This First

I am sorry I cannot devise a key by which to read this book, as well as a Key to the Calories, for sometimes you are to read the title headings and side explanations before the text. Other times you are supposed to read the text and then the headings. It really does not matter much as long as you read them both. Be sure to do that. They are clever. I wrote them myself.

I have been accused of trying to catch you coming and going, because I have included in my book the right methods of gaining weight, as well as those for losing weight. But this is not the reason--though I don't object to doing that little thing--the reason is that the lack of knowledge of foods is the foundation for both overweight and underweight.

I did want my publishers to get this out in a cheaper edition, thinking that more people could have it, and thus it would be doing more good; but they have convinced me that that idea was a false claim of my mortal mind, and that the more you paid for it, the more you would appreciate it. I have received many times, and without grumbling on my part, ten dollars for the same advice given in my office. Perhaps on this line of reasoning we should have ten dollars for the book. Those of you who think so may send the balance on through my publishers.

L.H.P.

Los Angeles, California June, 1918

CONTENTS

1 Preliminary Bout 11 2 Key to the Calories 23 3 Review and More Definitions 30 4 More Keys and More Calories 37 5 Vegetarianism vs. Meat Eating 54 6 The Deluded Ones--My Thin Friends 59 7 Exercise 69 8 At Last! How to Reduce 77 9 Autobiographical 88 10 Testimonials 96 11 An Apology and Some Amendments 98 12 Maintenance Diet and Conclusions 102 13 Three Years Later 106

Diet and Health

1

Preliminary Bout

Rule to Find Ideal Adult Net Weight

Multiply number of inches over 5 ft. in height by 5-1/2; add 110. For example: Height 5 ft. 7 in. without shoes.

7 x 5-1/2 = 38-1/2 + 110 ------- Ideal weight 148-1/2

If under 5 ft. multiply number of inches under 5 ft. by 5-1/2 and subtract from 110.

Are You Thin and Do You Want to Gain?

[Sidenote: Don't Read This]

Skip this chapter. It will not interest you in the least. I will come to you later. I am not particularly interested in you anyway, for I cannot get your point of view. How any one can want to be anything but thin is beyond my intelligence. However, knowing that there are such deluded individuals, I have been constrained to give you advice. You won't find it spontaneous nor from the heart, but if you follow my directions I will guarantee that you will gain; providing, of course, you have no organic trouble; and the chances are that by giving proper attention to your diet you will gain anyway, and maybe in passing lose your trouble. Who knows?

[Sidenote: Bad Business]

In war time it is a crime to hoard food, and fines and imprisonment have followed the expos?of such practices. Yet there are hundreds of thousands of individuals all over America who are hoarding food, and that one of the most precious of all foods! They have vast amounts of this valuable commodity stored away in their own anatomy.

[Illustration: contents noted]

Now fat individuals have always been considered a joke, but you are a joke no longer. Instead of being looked upon with friendly tolerance and amusement, you are now viewed with distrust, suspicion, and even aversion! How dare you hoard fat when our nation needs it? You don't dare to any longer. You never wanted to be fat anyway, but you did not know how to reduce, and it is proverbial how little you eat. Why, there is Mrs. Natty B. Slymm, who is beautifully thin, and she eats twice as much as you do, and does not gain an ounce. You know positively that eating has nothing to do with it, for one time you dieted, didn't eat a thing but what the doctor ordered, besides your regular meals, and you actually gained.

You are in despair about being anything but fat, and--! how you hate it. But cheer up. I will save you; yea, even as I have saved myself and many, many others, so will I save you.

[Sidenote: Spirituality vs. Materiality]

[Sidenote: A Long, Long Battle]

It is not in vain that all my life I have had to fight the too, too solid. Why, I can remember when I was a child I was always being consoled by being told that I would outgrow it, and that when I matured I would have some shape. Never can I tell pathetically "when I was married I weighed only one hundred eighteen, and look at me now." No, I was a delicate slip of one hundred and sixty-five when I was taken.

I never will tell you how much I have weighed, I am so thoroughly ashamed of it, but my normal weight is one hundred and fifty pounds, and at one time there was seventy pounds more of me than there is now, or has been since I knew how to control it. I was not so shameless as that very long, and as I look back upon that short period I feel like refunding the comfortable salary received as superintendent of an hospital; for I know I was only sixty-five per cent efficient, for efficiency decreases in direct proportion as excess weight increases. Everybody knows it.

The Meeting Is Now Open for Discussion

Jolly Mrs. Sheesasite has the floor and wants some questions answered. You know Mrs. Sheesasite; her husband recently bought her a pair of freight scales.

[Sidenote: Mrs. Sheesasite]

"Why is it, Doctor, that thin people can eat so much more than fat people and still not gain?"

[Sidenote: Me Answering]

"First: Thin people are usually more active than fat people and use up their food.

"Second: Thin people have been proved to radiate fifty per cent more heat per pound than fat people; in other words, fat people are regular fireless cookers! They hold the heat in, it cannot get out through the packing, and the food which is also contained therein goes merrily on with fiendish regularity, depositing itself as fat.

[Illustration: Fireless Cookers.]

"And there are baby fireless cookers and children fireless cookers. The same dietetic rules apply to them as to the adult."

"I recognize Mrs. Tiny Weyaton; then you, Mrs. Knott Little."

[Sidenote: Mrs. Weyaton]

"We have heard you say that fat people eat too much, and still we eat so little?"

[Sidenote: Me Again]

"Yes, you eat too much, no matter how little it is, even if it be only one bird-seed daily, if you store it away as fat. For, hearken; food, and food only (sometimes plus alcohol) maketh fat. Not water--not air--verily, nothing but food maketh fat. (And between you and me, Mrs. Weyaton, just confidential like--don't tell it--we know that the small appetite story is a myth.)"

[Sidenote: Mrs. Knott Little]

"But, Doctor, is it not true that some individuals inherit the tendency to be fat, and can not help it, no matter what they do?"

[Sidenote: Doctor]

"Answer to first part--Yes.

"Answer to second part--No! It is not true that they cannot help it; they have to work a little harder, that is all. It is true that being fat is a disease with some, due to imperfect working of the internal secretory glands, such as the thyroid, generative glands, etc.; but that is not true fat such as you have. Yours, and that of the other members who are interested, is due to overeating and underexercising.

[Sidenote: Not?]

"Those diseased individuals should be under the care of a physician. Probably the secretory glands are somewhat inactive or sluggish in the healthy fat individual. I use the word healthy here in contradistinction to the other type. In reality, individuals very much overweight are not really healthy, and they should also visit their physician."

"Yes, Mrs. Ima Gobbler?"

[Sidenote: Mrs. Ima Gobbler]

[Sidenote: Doctor Dear]

"But, Doctor dear, what's the use of dieting? I only get fatter after I stop."

(Answering delicate like, for I'm fond of her and she is sensitive):

"You fat--! You make me fatigued! You never diet long enough to get out of the fireless cooker class. If you did, you wouldn't."

"Is there anyone else who would like to be recognized? No?"

[Sidenote: Nothing That I Don't Know]

It is well. I will probably answer more as I go along, for there is nothing that I don't know or haven't studied or tried in the reducing line. I know everything you have to contend with--how you no sooner congratulate yourself on your will power, after you have dragged yourself by the window with an exposure of luscious fat chocolates with curlicues on their tummies, than another comes into view, and you have it all to go through with again, and how you finally succumb.

I hope sometime it will be a misdemeanor, punishable by imprisonment, to display candy as shamelessly as it is done.

Many fond parents think that candy causes worms. It doesn't, of course, unless it is contaminated with worm eggs, but, personally, I wish every time I ate a chocolate I would get a worm, then I would escape them. The chocolates, I mean. I will tell you more about worms when I discuss meat.

[Sidenote: Vampires]

[Sidenote: Malicious Animal Magnetism?]

I know how you go down to destruction for peanuts, with their awful fat content. It is terrible, the lure a peanut has for me. Do you suppose Mr. Darwin could explain that?

Perhaps I was a little too delicate like in my answer to Mrs. Gobbler's question,--What's the use of dieting, she only gets fatter after she stops?

So many ask me that question, with the further pathetic addition,--Will they always have to keep it up? And it ever irritates me.

The answer is,--Yes! You will always have to keep up dieting, just as you always have to keep up other things in life that make it worth living--being neat, being kind, being tender; reading, studying, loving.

You will not have to be nearly so strenuous after you get to normal; but you might as well recognize now, and accept it as a fact, that neither you nor anybody else will be able to eat beyond your needs without accumulating fat or disease, or both.

I love Billy Sunday's classical answer to the objection that his conversions were not permanent. He responded: "Neither is a bath!"

WHEN YOU START TO REDUCE you will have the following to combat:

[Sidenote: A Combat]

First: Your husband, who tells you that he does not like thin women. I almost hate my husband when I think how long he kept me under that delusion. Now, of course, I know all about his jealous disposition, and how he did not want me to be attractive.

[Illustration: Green!]

Second: Your sister, who says, "Goodness, Lou, but you look old today; you looked lots better as you were."

[Illustration: Sweet Peace]

Third: Your friends, who tell you that you are just right now; don't lose another pound! And other friends who tell you cheerful tales of people they have known who reduced, and who went into a decline, and finally died.

[Sidenote: To Avoid Slack in Your Neck, Double and Triple Chins, Massage Vigorously Up and Down, Not Crossways]

[Sidenote: I Am Interesting]

But you must not mind them. Smile, and tell them that you know all about it, and don't worry. Go serenely on your way, confident in your heart that you will look fully ten years younger when you get down to normal, no matter how you look in the interim. I don't see why women, and men, too, (secretly) worry so much about wrinkles. If the increased wrinkles on the face are accompanied by increased wrinkles in the gray matter, 'tis a consummation devoutly to be wished. I'm sure I am much more interesting with wrinkles than I was without. I am to myself, anyway.

However, you will not be any more wrinkled if you reduce gradually, as I advise, and keep up your exercises at least fifteen minutes daily.

[Sidenote: I Have a Beautiful Complexion]

[Sidenote: I Attended an Art School Six Months Once]

Take care of your face, alternate hot and cold water, glycerine one-quarter, rose water three-quarters, cold cream packs, massage gently, a little ice--you know what to do--you need not fear. You will not only look ten years younger and live twenty years longer--I assert it boldly--but your complexion and efficiency will be one hundred per cent better.

[Sidenote: Joy!]

If there is anything comparable to the joy of taking in your clothes, I have not experienced it. And when you find your corset coming closer and closer together (I advise a front lace, so this can be watched), and then the day you realize that you will have to stitch in a tuck or get a new one!

But don't be in a hurry to make your clothes smaller now. If they are loose they will show to the world that you are reducing. A fat person in a tight suit, unless it is perfectly new, should be interned.

[Sidenote: Food Only]

[Sidenote: Impossible]

I have said that food, and food only, causes fat. That gives you the cue to what you must do to get rid of it. No anti-fat medicines unless under the supervision of your scientific, educated physician. They are dangerous; most of them contain thyroid extract, arsenic, or mercury. Even the vendors of these harmful compounds in their advertisements are now saying to "stop harmful drugging," but urge you to adopt their particular delightful product, and, "without dieting or exercises, you will positively reduce," and so forth.

No drastic purges, no violent exercises, especially at first, and not too frequent nor prolonged Turkish baths. Epsom salts baths have little effect. If salts are used habitually internally, they are harmful. All of these are unscientific and unsuccessful, and the things they bring on are worse than the fat.

Now, if food is the only source of body substance, you see that you must study that question, and that is what I will give you--some lessons on foods and their values.

[Sidenote: Candy Cake, Pie, Rich Meats, Thick Gravy, Bread, Butter, Nuts, Ice Cream]

[Sidenote: Whipped Cream, Candied Sweet Potatoes]

Heretofore you have known only in a dumb, despairing sort of way that all the foods you like are fattening, and all the advice you read and hear is that you must avoid them as a pestilence. And you settle down to your joyless fatness, realizing that it is beyond human strength to do that forever, and that you would rather die young and fat, anyway, than to have nothing to eat all your life but a little meat, fish, and sloshy vegetables. Study on, and you will find the reason your favorite foods are fattening.

But cast off your dejection. You don't have to avoid them!

Eat what you like and grow thin? Yes; follow me. I know it will be an exertion, but you must persist and go through with it. Nothing in life worth while is attained without some effort. So begin now; it is the price of liberty.

Review

1. Give rule for normal weight.

2. How much excess food have you stored away?

3. Why more important than ever to reduce?

4. Why are fat individuals fireless cookers?

5. Give causes of excess fat.

NOTE: The Reviews which follow the chapters are important and the questions should be answered. To get the full benefit, Little Book must be studied, for it is the only authorized textbook of the "Watch Your Weights."

2

Key to the Calories

Some one page the thin? They come back here.

[Sidenote: Don't Skip This]

Definition to learn:

CALORIE; symbol C.; a heat unit and food value unit; is that amount of heat necessary to raise one pound of water 4 degrees Fahrenheit.

[Sidenote: Pronounced Kal'-o-ri]

There is a good deal of effort expended by many semi-educated individuals to discredit the knowledge of calories, saying that it is a foolish food science, a fallacy, a fetish, and so forth.

They reason, or rather say, that because there are no calories in some of the very vital elements of foods--the vitamines and the mineral salts--therefore it is not necessary to know about them. They further argue that their grandfathers never heard of calories and they got along all right. That grandfather argument always enrages my mortal mind.

[Sidenote: A Unit of Measure]

Now you know that a calorie is a unit of measuring heat and food. It is not heat, not food; simply a unit of measure. And as food is of supreme importance, certainly a knowledge of how it should be measured is also of supreme importance.

[Sidenote: Yes, They Are Kosher]

You should know and also use the word calorie as frequently, or more frequently, than you use the words foot, yard, quart, gallon, and so forth, as measures of length and of liquids. Hereafter you are going to eat calories of food. Instead of saying one slice of bread, or a piece of pie, you will say 100 Calories of bread, 350 Calories of pie.

The following is the way the calorie is determined:

An apparatus known as the bomb calorimeter has two chambers, the inner, which contains the dry food to be burned, say a definite amount of sugar, and an outer, which is filled with water. The food is ignited with an electric connection and burned. This heat is transferred to the water. When one pound of water is raised 4 degrees Fahrenheit, the amount of heat used is arbitrarily chosen as the unit of heat, and is called the Calorie.

Food burned (oxydized) in the body has been proved to give off approximately the same amount of heat or energy as when burned in the calorimeter.

[Sidenote: Approximate Measures]

1 oz. Fat = 275 C. --about 255 in the body.

1 oz. Protein (dry) = 120 C. --about 113 in the body.

1 oz. Carbohydrates (dry) = 120 C. --about 113 in the body.

(ROSE.)

Can you see now why fats are valuable? Why they make fat more than any other food? They give off more than two and one-fourth times as much heat, or energy, as the other foods.

[Sidenote: See Next Chapter for Definitions]

Notice that protein and carbohydrates have the same food value as to heat or energy, each 113 Calories to the dry ounce. However, they are not interchangeable; that is, carbohydrates will not take the place of protein for protein is absolutely necessary to build and repair tissue, and carbohydrates cannot do that. But fats and carbohydrates are interchangeable as fuel or energy foods.

Calories Needed per Day for Normal Individuals

[Sidenote: Business of Growing]

This depends upon age, weight, and physical activities; the baby and the growing child needing many more calories per pound per day than the adult, who has to supply only his energy and repair needs. The aged require still less than the young adult. As to weight; I have told you why overweight individuals need so little. As to physical activities; the more active, obviously the more calories needed, for every movement consumes calories.

[Sidenote: Many Know Nothing of This]

The Maine lumbermen, for instance, while working during the winter months, consume from 5000 to 8000 Calories per day. But they do a tremendous amount of physical work.

Mental work does not require added nourishment. This has been proved, and if an excess be taken over what is needed at rest (if considerable exercise is not taken while doing the mental work) the work is not so well done.

[Sidenote: Calories Required for Normal]

Per pound per day

Infants require 40-50 C. Growing Children 30-40 C. Adults (depending upon activity) 15-20 C. Old age requires 15 or less C.

In Round Numbers for the Day

Child 2-6 1000 to 1600 C. per day Child 6-12 1600 to 2500 C. per day Youth 12-18 2500 to 3000 C. per day

[Sidenote: Growth Demands]

(Remember that in general the boy needs as much as his father, and the girl as much as her mother.)

MAN (per day):

At rest 1800 to 2000 C. Sedentary 2200 to 2800 C. Working 3500 to 4000 C.

WOMAN (per day):

At rest 1600 to 1800 C. Sedentary occupations (bookkeeper, etc.) 2000 to 2200 C. Occupations involving standing, walking, or manual labor (general housekeeping, etc.) 2200 to 2500 C. Occupations requiring strength (laundress, etc.) 2500 to 3000 C. (ROSE.)

Example of Finding Number of Calories Needed

1. Determine normal weight by rule.

2. Multiply normal weight by number of calories needed per pound per day.

For example, say you weigh 220 or 125 lbs., but by the rule for your height your weight should be 150 lbs.; then 150 would be the number you would use.

[Sidenote: Work Out Your Requirements]

By the rule I have given, adults require 15-20 Calories per pound per day, depending upon activity. For example, if you have no physical activities, then take the lowest figure, 15. 150x15--2250. Therefore your requirement, if your weight should be 150, is 2250 Calories per day.

Now, if you want to lose, cut down 500-1000 Calories per day from that.

Five hundred Calories equal approximately 2 ounces of fat. Two ounces per day would be about 4 pounds per month, or 48 pounds per year. Cutting out 1000 Calories per day would equal a reduction of approximately 8 pounds per month, or 96 pounds per year. These pounds you can absolutely lose by having a knowledge of food values (calories) and regulating your intake accordingly. You can now see the importance of a knowledge of calories.

[Sidenote: 1 lb. fat 4000 C 1/2 lb. fat 2000 C 1/4 lb. fat 1000 C 1/8 lb. fat 500 C]

If you want to gain, add gradually 500-1000 Calories per day.

Review

1. Define Calorie, and tell how determined.

2. How many C. in 1 oz. fat? of carbohydrates? of protein?

3. Why are fats so fattening?

4. How many C. per day do you require? do mental workers?

5. Upon what do C. needed per day for normal individuals depend? Discuss.

Review and More Definitions

[Sidenote: This Is Dry but Important]

FOOD: That which taken into the body builds and repairs tissue and yields energy in heat and muscular power.

[Sidenote: Approx. %'s if Normal]

CLASSES OF FOOD:

1. Protein, 18% of body weight. 2. Fats, 16% of body weight. 3.

Carbohydrates, 1% of body weight. 4. Mineral matter, 5% of body weight. 5. Vitamines. 6. Water, 60% of body weight.

[Sidenote: Nitrogenous Food Compounds]

PROTEIN: Builds tissue, repairs waste, yields energy, and may help store fat. One-half, at least, of your protein should be from the vegetable kingdom.

A large percentage of protein is contained in

Eggs Meat Fowl Fish Nuts Milk Cheese Gluten of Wheat Legumes (beans, peas, lentils, peanuts, etc.)

[Sidenote: Protein 113 C. Per Oz.]

There is about one-fourth ounce protein in

1 egg 1 glass milk (skim, butter, or whole) 1-1/2 oz. lean meat, or fish or fowl 1 oz. (1-1/5 cu. in.) whole milk cheese 2 slices of bread, 3-1/2 x 3-1/2 x 1/2 (white, whole wheat, corn, etc.) 3 heaping tablespoonfuls canned baked beans or lima beans 17 peanuts

[Sidenote: 255 C. Per Oz.]

FATS: Yield energy and are stored as fat.

Animal Fat: Cream, Butter, Lard

Oils: Cottonseed, Olive Almonds, Peanuts, Walnuts Chocolate, etc.

[Sidenote: 113 C. Per Oz.]

CARBOHYDRATES: Yield energy and are stored as fat.

Sugars (candy, honey, syrup, sweet fruits)

Starches (breads, cereals, potatoes, corn, legumes, nuts)

Vegetable fibre, or cellulose

MINERAL MATTER: Shares in forming bones and teeth, and is necessary for proper functioning.

Carbon Lime Sodium Potassium, Sulphur Iron Phosphorus Etc.

[Sidenote: Whole Grain Products Not Devitalized]

These elements are contained largely in the outer coatings of grains, fruits, and vegetables, and in animal foods and their products. Do not pare potatoes before cooking. Cook vegetables in a small amount of water, saving the water for soups and sauces.

WATER: The universal solvent, absolutely necessary for life.

Contained in purest form in all vegetables and fruits. The average person needs, in addition, from three to five pints taken as a drink. If not sure of the purity, boil. Do not drink while food is in the mouth.

[Sidenote: Absolutely Necessary for Growth]

VITAMINES: Health preservers. Vital substances necessary for growth. The chemistry of these products is at present not thoroughly understood, but their importance has been demonstrated by experiments (not torture) on animals. By this work we know that diseases like beri-beri, scurvy, rickets, and probably pellagra, are due to a lack of these vital elements in the food, and from that fact these are called "deficiency" diseases.

[Sidenote: Guinea Pigs vs. Babies]

Of course I realize that nations can be saved from horrible diseases, and hundreds and thousands of babies saved from death, through this experimentation on a few guinea pigs and other animals; but what is the life of a baby compared with the happiness of a guinea pig? Down with animal experimentation! Let us do everything in our power to hamper scientific work of this kind. We are giving up our husbands, fathers, sons, perhaps to die, for the cause of humanity, but a guinea pig! Horrors!

It has been found that the vitamines, like the minerals, are most abundant in the outer coverings and the germ of grains, and in fruits and vegetables. They are also present in fresh milk, butter, meat and eggs. Babies fed pasteurized or boiled milk should have fruit juices and vegetable purees early. Begin with one-half teaspoonful, well diluted, and gradually increase the feeding to an ounce or more between meals once or twice daily.

Most animal fats have the vitamines, but vegetable fats are deficient in them. That is the reason cod liver oil is better for some therapeutic uses than olive oil.

[Sidenote: Balanced Diet]

BALANCED DIET: Should contain

10-15% Protein (children may need more) 25-30% Fat 60-65% Carbohydrates

[Sidenote: To Get the Elements Necessary for Health]

For example, suppose you are a fairly active woman and need 2500 calories per day. Then for a balanced diet you would need:

10% Protein, or 250 C. 25% Fat, or 625 C. 65% Carbohydrates 1625 C. ------- 2500 C.

250 C. of P. = 2-1/5 oz. dry protein (250 ?113 = 2-1/5, approximately) 625 C. of F. = 2-1/2 oz. of fat (625 ?255 = 2-1/2, approximately) 1625 C. of CH. = 14-1/2 oz. dry carbohydrates (1625 ?113 = 14-1/2, approximately)

Two and one-fifth ounces dry protein equals the approximate amount of protein in 10 ounces lean meat, fish, or fowl, or 9 ounces cheese, or 9 eggs. (You should not take all of your proteins in any of these single forms.) Two and one-half ounces fat equals approximately 5 pats of butter.

[Sidenote: If Appetite Not Perverted]

But listen! You don't have to bother with all this fussy stuff. Be careful not to over-or under-eat of the proteins, and your tastes will be a fair standard for the rest. You should remember that a balanced diet contains some of all these foods, in about the proportions given, and that, while watery vegetables and fruits contain very few calories, they contain very important mineral salts, vitamines, and cellulose. The latter is good for the daily scrub of the intestinal tract.

[Sidenote: A Pretty Nearly Universal Error]

CONSTIPATION is many times caused by a too concentrated diet, or one containing too little roughage. It has also been discovered that some individuals who are troubled with faulty elimination digest this cellulose, and only the more resistant, like bran, is not absorbed. For those, the Japanese seaweed called agaragar in the laboratory, but more familiarly known as agar by the layman, is excellent. The most industrious digestive tract apparently can not digest that. It has the further property of absorbing a large amount of water, thus increasing its bulk.

[Sidenote: C.S.]

[Sidenote: Have Enough Water, Else You'll Choke to Death. I Did Once]

Mineral oils (refined paraffine) also are not absorbable, and they act with benefit in some cases. About the worst thing to do, in general, is to take physics constantly. These are not physics, however; they act mechanically. Even the C.S. (common-sense?) individual can take these. The agar may be taken two or three heaping teaspoonfuls in a large glass of water before retiring, or in the morning before breakfast, or in lieu of 4 o'clock tea. Drink it down rapidly--for goodness' sake, don't try to chew it.

Mineral oil will make fine mayonnaise dressing. It has little or no food value, so the constipated overweight individual may indulge freely. For faulty elimination, then--

1. Correct diet.

2. Exercise--especially brisk walking.

3. Regularity of habit.

4. Possibly the addition of bran, agar, or mineral oils.

5. Sweet disposition. Mean people are always constipated.

Review

1. Give classes of food, with examples of each.

2. What are vitamines? How importance discovered?

3. Where most abundant?

4. What is a balanced diet?

5. What should be done for faulty elimination?

4

More Keys and More Calories

[Sidenote: List of Foods to Follow]

The following list probably does not contain all of the foods you might like and want to know about, but from those named you can judge of the food value of others. In general, the caloric value, and therefore the fattening value, depends upon the amount of fat and the degree of concentration.

[Sidenote: Important]

But remember this point: Any food eaten beyond what your system requires for its energy, growth, and repair, is fattening, or is an irritant, or both.

[Sidenote: A Moderate Sized Chocolate Cream]

If a food contains much fat, you will know that it is high in food value, for fat has two and one-quarter times the caloric value that proteins and carbohydrates have. Dry foods are high in value, for they are concentrated and contain little water. Compare the quantity of two heaping teaspoonfuls of sugar, a concentrated food, and one and one-half pounds of lettuce, a watery vegetable, each having the same caloric value. A moderate sized chocolate cream is not only concentrated but has considerable fat in the chocolate.

[Sidenote: Enuf Sed]

It is not necessary to know accurately the caloric values. In fact, authorities differ in some of their computations. The list is not mathematically correct, but it will give you a good idea of the relative values, and is accurate enough for our purposes. I have purposely given round numbers, where possible, in order to make them more easily remembered.

In reckoning made dishes, such as puddings and sauces, you must compute the different ingredients approximately. About how much sugar it has, how much fat to the dish, and so on. In reckoning any food, if you are reducing, give it the benefit of the doubt on the high count; and if trying to gain, count it low.

It is well, if you are much overweight or underweight, to have some of these foods that are given weighed, so that you can judge approximately what your servings will total.

[Sidenote: A Mixture]

A mixture of foods should be used, in order to get the different elements which are necessary for the human machine. It is not wholesome to have many foods at a meal; but the menu should be varied from day to day.

Any regimen which does not allow some carbohydrates and fats for the fuel foods is injurious if persisted in for a length of time.

[Sidenote: Thoroughly Masticate Everything]

As to harmful combinations; there are not many, and if your food is thoroughly masticated you need not concern yourself very much about them. However, if you find a food disagrees with you, or that certain combinations disagree, do not try to use them. Underweight individuals sometimes have to train their digestive tracts for some of the foods they need.

Coffee, tea and other mild stimulants are not harmful to the majority; but, like everything else, in excess they will cause ill health. Alcoholic drinks make the fat fatter and the thin thinner, and both more feeble mentally.

[Sidenote: I Love Her]

I hope I have stimulated you to an interest in dietetics. There are many books which go into the subject much more deeply. I recommend, especially, "The Home Dietitian," written by my beloved colleague and classmate, Dr. Belle Wood-Comstock.

Others I have read that are especially suitable for the home are "Feeding the Family," by Mary Schwartz Rose, and "Dietary Computer," by Pope. There are doubtless many other good ones. The Department of Agriculture publishes free bulletins on the subject. Farmers' Bulletin No. 142, by Atwater, is very comprehensive.

Other authorities I have consulted are Lusk, Friedenwald and Ruhr 鋒, Gautier, Sherman, Buttner, Locke and Von Noorden.

Measuring Table

1 teaspoon (tsp.) fluid 1/6 oz. 1 dessertspoon (tsp.) 1/3 oz. 1 tablespoon (tbsp.) 1/2 oz. 1 ordinary cup 8 oz. 1 ordinary glass 8 oz. Average helping a.h.

One Hundred Calorie Portions and Average Helpings

(Approximate Measures)

(ATWATER, LOCKE, ROSE)

MEATS

Beefsteak, lean round..............2 oz. 100 C. A.h....... 3-1/2 oz., 185 C. Beefsteak, tenderloin..............1 oz. 100 C. A.h.................. 285 C. Beef, roast, very lean.............3 oz. 100 C. A.h.................. 150 C.

Chicken, roast..................1-2/3oz. 100 C. 1 slice.............. 180 C. Frankfurters, 1 sausage............1 oz. 100 C. Chops, lamb or mutton..........1-1/2 oz. 100 C. Average chops.... 150-300 C.

Pork: Bacon, crisp...................1/2 oz. 100 C. 1 small slice, crisp 25 C. Chop........................1-1/2 oz. 100 C. Medium..........160-300 C. Ham, boiled................1-1/3 oz. 100 C. A.h..........3 oz., 250 C. Ham, fried.................3/4 oz. 100 C. A.h........3 oz., 400 C. Sausage........................1 oz. 100 C. 1 small, crisp.......60 C. Turkey.......................1-1/3 oz. 100 C. A.h........3-1/3 oz., 260 C.

[Sidenote: Fish Boiled or Broiled]

FISH

Fish, Lean, Cod, Halibut...........3 oz. 100 C. A.h........... 4 oz., 135 C. Fish, fat, salmon, sardines ...1 1/2 oz. 100 C. A.h.......... 4 oz., 260 C. Lobster...........................4 oz. 100 C. A.h.............. 100 C. Oysters....................... 12 100 C. 1 oyster.............. 8 C. Clams, long...................... 8 100 C. 1 clam............... 12 C.

SOUPS

Cream soups, average...............3 oz. 100 C. A.h.......... 4 oz., 125 C. Consomm 閎, no fat.................30 oz. 100 C. A.h.......... 4 oz., 15 C.

DAIRY PRODUCTS AND EGGS

Butter, 1 level tbsp. scant .... 1/2 oz. 100 C. 1 ball............... 120 C. Cheese (American, Roquefort, Swiss, etc.)..... 1-1/8 cu. in 3/4 oz. 100 C. Cottage Cheese.................. 3 oz. 100 C. A.h................ 100 C. Whole Milk..................... 5 oz. 100 C. 1 glass.............. 160 C. Skim Milk..................... 10 oz. 100 C. 1 glass............... 80 C. Malted Milk (dry)............1 h. tbsp. 100 C. Buttermilk, natural.............. 10 oz. 100 C. 1

glass............. 80 C. Koumiss........................... 6 oz. 100 C. 1 glass............. 130 C. Condensed, unsweetened............ 2 oz. 100 C. 1 tbsp............... 35 C. Condensed, sweetened, 1-1/4 tbsp....... 100 C. Cream, average................1-1/3 oz. 100 C. 1 tbsp............... 50 C. Cream, whipped................ 1-1/3 oz. 100 C. 1 h. tbsp............ 100 C. Eggs, 1 large..................... 1 100 C. Average egg........... 80 C. Boiled or poached; if fried, C. depend upon fat adhering.

VEGETABLES

When not otherwise indicated, the method of cooking is by boiling. The caloric value of sauces served with them not included.

Asparagus, large stalks........... 20 100 C. 1 stalk............... 5 C. Beets........................... 1 lb. 100 C. 2 h. tbsp............ 30 C. Beans, Baked, home............1-1/2 oz. 100 C. 3 h. tbsp............ 300 C. Beans, Baked, canned...........2-1/2 oz. 100 C. 3 h. tbsp............ 150 C. Beans, Lima...................... 3 oz. 100 C. 3 h. tbsp............ 130 C. Beans, String.................... 1 lb. 100 C. 2 h. tbsp............ 15 C. Cabbage........................ 1-1/2 lb. 100 C. 3 h. tbsp............. 10 C. Carrots........................... 1 lb. 100 C. 3 h. tbsp............ 20 C. Cauliflower....................... 1 lb. 100 C. 3 h. tbsp............ 20 C. Celery, uncooked.................. 1 lb. 100 C. 6 stalks............... 15 C. Corn, canned.................. 3-1/3 oz. 100 C. 2 h. tbsp............ 100 C. Corn, green, 1 ear........... 3-1/3 oz. 100 C. Medium size. Cucumber...................... 1-1/2 lb. 100 C. 10 to 12 thin slices.. 10 C. Lettuce..................... 1-1/2 lb. 100 C. A.h................ 5-10 C. Mushrooms........................ 8 oz. 100 C. Onions, 2 large.................. 8 oz. 100 C. Parsnips....................... 8 oz. 100 C. A.h............ 2 oz., 25 C. Peas, green..................... 3 oz. 100 C. A.h., 3 h. tbsp...... 100 C. Potatoes, sweet............... 1-1/2 oz. 100 C. 1 medium............. 200 C. Potatoes, white................ 3 oz. 100 C. 1 medium............. 100 C. Potato Chips......scant........... 1 oz. 100 C. A.h., 8-10 pieces.... 100 C. Radishes........................ 1 lb. 100 C. A.h., 6 red button.... 15 C. Spinach..................... 1-1/2 lb. 100 C. A.h., 1/2 cup......... 25 C. Squash...................... 1 lb. 100 C. A.h., 2h. tbsp........ 25 C. Tomatoes..................... 1 lb. 100 C. A.h., 1 large......... 50 C.

Turnips................... 1 lb. 100 C. A.h., 2 h. tbsp....... 25 C.

FRUITS

Apple........................ 7 oz. 100 C. 1 average size......... 50 C.
Banana..................... 5 oz. 100 C. 1 small............... 100 C.
Berries............average....... 5 oz. 100 C. 1 small cup......... 100 C.
Cantaloupe.................. 1 lb. 100 C. A.h., 1/2 melon....... 100 C.
Cherries.................... 5 oz. 100 C. A.h., 1 small cup..... 100 C.
Grapes..................... 5 oz. 100 C. A.h., 1 small bunch... 100 C. Lemons (5 oz. each).............. 2 100 C. They won't make you thin. Average size.......... 30 C. Oranges (9 oz. each).............. 1 100 C. Peaches (5 oz. each)............. 2 100 C. Average size.......... 50 C. Pears (6 oz. each)................ 1 100 C. Average size.......... 90 C. Pineapple, fresh................. 7 oz. 100 C. 2 slices, 1 in. thick. 100 C. Plums, large..................... 3 or 4 100 C. 1 plum............... 30 C. Watermelon................... 1-1/2 lb. 100 C. Large slice........... 15 C. Dates (dry), large............... 3-4 100 C. 1 large............... 25 C. Figs (dry), large............... 1-1/2 100 C. 1 large............... 65 C. Prunes (dry), large............. 3 100 C. 1 large............... 35 C. Stewed, 4 medium, with 4 tbsp. juice....... 200 C.

BREAD AND CRACKERS

Brown Bread, 1 slice, 3 in. in diam., 3/4 in. thick 100 C. Corn Bread, 3 x 2 x 3/4 1-1/2 oz. 100 C. Victory Bread, 1 slice, 3 x 4 x 1/2 in. 100 C.

White, gluten, rye, whole wheat, etc., practically same caloric value per same weight. There is so little difference between the caloric value of gluten bread and other breads that it is not necessary for reducing to try to get it. (Toasted bread has the same caloric value that it had before toasting. It is more easily digested, but just as fattening. Advised, however, because it makes you chew.)

1 French or Vienna roll 100 C. Zweiback 3/4 oz. 100 C. 1 slice, 3-1/4 x 1-1/4 x 1/2 in., 35 C. Graham Crackers 3 100 C. 1 c., 3 in. sq. 35 C. Oyster Crackers 24

100 C. Soda Crackers 4 100 C. 1 c. 25 C. Pretzels 5 100 C. 1 p. 20 C.

BREAKFAST FOODS, ETC.

Farina or Cream of Wheat 6 oz. 100 C. 2 h. tbsp 60 C. Force 1 oz. 100 C. 5 h. tbsp 65 C. Grapenuts scant 1 oz. 100 C. 2 tbsp 100 C. Griddle Cakes, 4-1/2 in. in diam. 100 C. A.h., 3 cakes 300 C. (This does not include butter and syrup, remember.) Hominy 4 oz. 100 C. 2 h. tbsp 85 C. Macaroni, plain 4 oz. 100 C. 2 h. tbsp 90 C. Macaroni and cheese (depends on amt. cheese) 2 h. tbsp 200-300 C. Muffin, average 3/4 m. 100 C. 1 muffin 125 C. Oatmeal 5 oz. 100 C. 1 small cup 100 C. Puffed Rice 1 oz. 100 C. 5 h. tbsp 50 C. Popcorn (cups) 1-1/2 100 C. A.h. depends on butter added. Rice, boiled 4 oz. 100 C. 1/2 cup 100 C. Shredded Wheat Biscuit 1 100 C. Triscuits (2) 100 C. Waffles scant 1/2 w. 100 C. 1 waffle 225 C.

CANDY, PASTRIES AND SWEETS

Chocolate creams, medium. 1 100 C. Chocolate, 1 lb 2880 C. Cherries, candied 10 100 C. Cup Custard, 1/3 cup 100 C. Chocolate Nut Caramels 1 x 1 x 4/5 in. 100 C. Other candies, reckon sugar, nuts, etc. Cookies, plain, diam. 3 in. 2 100 C. 1 cookie 50 C. If raisins or nuts in them, count extra. Doughnut scant 2/3 100 C. 1 average size 160 C. Ginger-snap 5 100 C. 1 gingersnap 20 C. Honey h. tbsp. 1 100 C. Thick syrups approximately the same. Ladyfingers scant 1 oz. 100 C. 1 ladyfinger 35-50 C. Macaroons 2 100 C. 1 macaroon 50 C. Pie with top crust, about 1/4 ordinary slice, or 1-1/4 in. 100 C. A.h., 1/6 pie 350 C. Pie without top crust, 2 in. 100 C. Custard, lemon, squash, etc. A.h., 1/6 pie. 250-300 C. Puddings, average cup 1/4 100 C. A.h. 200-350 C. Depends upon richness. Ice Cream h. tbsp. 1 100 C. A.h. 200-350 C. Depends upon richness. Cakes 1 oz. 100 C. A.h. 200-350 C. Depends upon size, icing, fruit, nuts, etc.; compute approximately. Sugar cubes 3 100 C. Granulated h. tsp. 2 100 C.

Saccharine, a coal tar product 300 to 500 times sweeter than sugar, but of no food value. Not advisable to use habitually. Better learn to like things unsweetened--it can be done.

CONDIMENTS AND SAUCES

Mayonnaise m. tbsp. 1 100 C. A.h. 200 C. Olive oil and other oils. dsp. 1 100 C. Olives, green or ripe 6-8 100 C. 1 olive 10-15 C. Tomato Catsup 6 oz. 100 C. 1 tbsp. 10 C. Thick Gravies tbsp. 3 100 C.

NUTS

Almonds, large 10 100 C. 1 almond 10 C. Brazil, large 2-1/2 100 C. 1 Brazil nut 45 C. Chestnuts, small 20 100 C. 1 chestnut 5 C. Peanuts, large double 10 100 C. 1 bag 250-300 C. Pecans, large 5 100 C. 1 pecan 20 C. Walnuts, large 3-1/3 100 C. 1 walnut 30 C. Cocoanut, prepared 1/2 oz. 100 C. Peanut Butter 2-1/2 tsp. 100 C.

Key to Key

[Sidenote: Remember This]

If you will remember the following portions of food, you will have a standard by which to compute your servings:

Lean Meat: a piece 3 x 2 x 1/2 (2 oz.) 100 C. Now if your serving of meat or fish is fat, mentally cut in two for same value. If very lean, you should add a little. White Bread: slice 3 x 4x 1/2 100 C. Compute other breads by this. Butter: 1 scant tablespoonful 100 C. Sugar: 1 heaping teaspoonful 50 C. Potatoes: 1 medium, boiled or baked. 100 C. Watery Vegetables: 1 helping 15-35 C.

If food is fried, or butter, oil, or cream sauces are added, the C. value increases markedly.

Review

1. Why is a mixture of foods necessary?

2. Give the caloric value of the following: 1 glass of milk, skim; buttermilk; 10 chocolate creams; 1 bag peanuts; 1 pat butter; 1 piece pie.

3. Name foods low in caloric value. Why are they valuable?

4. How many calories of bread and butter do you daily consume?

5. Reckon your usual caloric intake. How much of it is in excess of your needs?

6. Memorize caloric value of foods you are fond of.

This Table of Foods, With the C Given Per Oz. Will Help You

The caloric value of pure fat is 255 C per oz., dry starches and sugars (carbohydrates), and protein (the meat element), is 113. This means fats are 2-1/4 times more fattening than other foods. Most foods contain considerable water, so the following is an approximate table of foods 'as is.' I have given round numbers in the table so you can more easily remember them. Memorize it.

Calories per oz.

Fats 255 Nuts, edible part 200 Sugar 115 Cream cheese 110 Cottage cheese (no fat) 30 Breads 75 Lean meats 50 Lean fish 35 Eggs (per oz.) 40 Milk, whole 20 Milk, skim and buttermilk (no fat) 10 Milk, condensed, sweet 100 Milk, condensed, unsweet. 50 Cream, thin 60 Cream, thick 110 Fruits: Dried 100 Sweet 25 Acid 15 Vegetables: Potatoes, plain (oz.) 30 Cooked Legumes, (peas, beans, etc.) 20-35 Watery and leafy 5-15

Vegetarianism vs. Meat Eating

[Sidenote: Protein]

As protein is the only food which builds and repairs tissue, it is the food which has caused the most controversy.

First: As to the amount needed.

Second: As to whether animal flesh protein is necessary.

[Sidenote: Chittenden]

AMOUNT NEEDED: It was thought for many years that 150 grams or 5 ounces of dry protein (equivalent to about 1-1/2 pounds lean meat) per day was necessary. But experiments of Chittenden and others have proved that considerably less is sufficient, and that the health is improved if less is taken.

Chittenden's standard is 50 grams, or 1-2/3 ounces, dry protein (equivalent to 1/2 pound meat per day). This is considered by many as insufficient. A variation from 1-2/3 to 3 ounces dry protein per day will give a safe range. (ROSE.)

[Sidenote: Approx. 240 to 360 C Per Day]

The amount of protein needed is comparatively independent of the amount of physical exertion, thus differing from the purely fuel foods, carbohydrates and fats, which should vary in direct proportion to the amount of physical exertion. In general, 10 to 15 per cent of the total calories per day should be taken as protein. An excess is undoubtedly irritant to the kidneys, blood vessels, and other organs, and if too little is taken the body tissues will suffer.

Not all of the protein should be taken in the form of animal protein; at least one-half should be taken from the vegetable kingdom.

Animal Flesh Protein

[Sidenote: Necessary?]

The following are a few of the chief reasons given by those who object to its use:

[Sidenote: The Negative Side]

First: The animal has just as much right to life, liberty, and pursuit of happiness as we have.

Second: They may be diseased, and there is the possibility of their containing animal parasites, such as tapeworms and trichin? I would like to tell you more about worms, they are so interesting, but He says not to try to tell all I know in this little book; that maybe he will let me write another sometime, although it is a terrible strain on him, and that I have given enough of the family history, anyway.

[Sidenote: Some Word]

Third: The tissues of animals contain excrementitious material, which may cause excess acidity, raise the blood pressure, and so forth.

Fourth: More apt to putrefy and thus give ptomaine poisoning.

Fifth: Makes the disposition more vicious.

(Honest,--animals eating meat exclusively are more vicious.)

[Sidenote: The Affirmative Side]

Those who believe that animal protein should be eaten answer these points as follows:

First: Survival of the fittest.

Second: If you give decent support to your health departments they can furnish enough inspectors to prevent the marketing of diseased meat; and if some should slip through, if you thoroughly bake, boil, or fry your animal parasites they will lose their pep.

Third: Most of the harmful products are destroyed by the intestines and liver.

Fourth: True, but see that you get good meat, and don't eat it in excess.

Fifth: Unanswerable--to be proved later by personal experiments.

In addition, they say that animal protein is more easily digested, that 97 per cent is assimilated because it is animal, and so it is much more to be desired, especially by children and convalescents; that vegetable protein is enclosed in cellulose, and only 65 to 75 per cent is used by the system; thus the diet is apt to be too bulky if the proper amount is taken.

[Sidenote: Strong Vegetarians]

It has been proved, however, by several endurance tests, that the vegetarian contestants had more strength and greater endurance than their meat-eating competitors, so there is no reason why we should be worried by one or two, or even more, meatless days, especially when animal product protein, such as milk, eggs, cheese, and the vegetable proteins, as in the legumes and the nuts, are available.

[Sidenote: A Confession]

I confess that for quite a while after studying vegetarian books I took a dislike to meat, but now I am in the comfortable state described by Benjamin Franklin in his autobiography. It seems that he had been converted to vegetarianism and had decided that he never again would eat the flesh of animals that had been ruthlessly slaughtered, when they so little deserved that fate.

But he was exceedingly fond of fish, and while on a fishing party, as some fish were being fried, he found they did smell most admirably well, and he was greatly torn between his desire and his principle. Finally he remembered that when the fish were opened he saw some smaller fish in their stomachs, and he decided that if they could eat each other he could eat them.

[Sidenote: Most Noted Picture of B. Franklin Extant]

Protein Calories in 100 C Portions of Food

In 100 C's Bread, 1 slice, (W.W. the highest) 12 to 16 C's P In 100 C's Cooked Cereals, 1 sm. cup, (oatmeal highest) 10 to 18 C's P In 100 C's Rice, 1 small cup 10 C's P In 100 C's Macaroni, 1 small cup 15 C's P In 100 C's Whole milk, 5 oz. 20 C's P In 100 C's Skim and buttermilk, 10 oz. 35 C's P In 100 C's Cheese, 3 heaping tbsp. Cottage cheese 75 C's P In 100 C's Eggs 1-1/3 36 C's P In 100 C's Meat or fish, Very lean 2-3 oz. 50 to 75 C's P In 100 C's Nuts, peanuts, almonds, walnuts. Peanuts the highest 10 to 20 C's P In 100 C's Beans 1/3 cup average 20 C's P In 100 C's Green peas 3/4 cup average 28 C's P In 100 C's Corn 1/3 cup average 12 C's P In 100 C's Onions 3 to 4 medium 12 C's P In 100 C's Potato 1 medium 12 C's P In 100 C's Tomatoes 1 lb 15 C's P In 100 C's Fresh fruits: berries, currants, rhubarb 10 C's P Others 2 to 5 C's P

The Deluded Ones--My Thin Friends

[Sidenote: What!]

I am going to sandwich you in between the food calories and my fat friends, and maybe you can absorb some of them. In the first chapter, you remember, I said I was not particularly interested in you, but I have changed my mind, and I will treat you tenderly and carefully. I will have to preach a little bit first, but I don't mind that; I love to reform people--Yes, you need reforming!

The first thing many of you have to do is to learn to accept the trivial annoyances and small misfits of life as a matter of course, for to give them attention beyond their deserts is to wear the web of your life to the warp.

Elbert Hubbard never said anything better than that. Have that reproduced in motto form and put it on your bureau, and repeat it fifty times daily.

[Sidenote: Good Philosophy]

Adopt my philosophy. If I have a trivial annoyance I analyze it carefully. Was I to blame? Yes? All right, I am glad, because then I can see that it will not happen again, so I stop worrying. If I am not to blame, if I could not help it in the least, well, then I don't worry about it, for that will not help it any, and I wasn't to blame! If it bobs up in my mind again, I say: "Now, look here, you annoyance, I have given you all the attention you deserve; avaunt, depart, get out!"

[Sidenote: Simple]

Now, how is this philosophy going to help you gain?

[Sidenote: Lost Calories]

When you worry needlessly, notice how tense your muscles are. You are exercising them all of the time and using hundreds of calories of energy. You raise your blood pressure, the internal secretory glands may overact (re-read what I have said about these glands in the fat people), and thus many more calories are used. The intestinal secretions do not flow so freely, you have indigestion and do not assimilate your food, and thus hundreds more calories are lost.

It certainly is impossible to gain unless your food is assimilated.

[Sidenote: Develop Poise]

So the first thing you have to learn is this mental control and to relax. Remember that word, relax. After you are better nourished your nervous system will not be on hair-trigger tension, and it will be easier for you.

[Sidenote: No Pain In Matter; No Matter In Pain Why Worry?]

If you are ill in mind or body, remember that it is natural to be well, and that within your body nature has stored the most wonderful forces which are always tending towards the normal, or health, if not obstructed or hindered.

Nature sometimes needs help to stimulate those forces, or to reinforce them, or to remove obstructions. This is where the physician comes in. But you yourself can aid nature the most by realizing that nature is health and it is normal to be well. By so doing, all of your organs function better and you are restored to normal more rapidly.

[Sidenote: Sleep]

[Sidenote: Fresh Air]

Second: It is very important to have enough sleep. Dr. Richard Cabot says that probably resistance is lowered as much by lack of sufficient sleep as by any other factor, and that all you can soak into your system in twenty-four hours is not too much. Don't forget the fresh air.

You generally suffer from sleeplessness, I believe. The overweights are always advised not to sleep too much. They will find while reducing that they won't want to sleep so much, anyway. They will like to stay awake--they feel so much happier.

[Sidenote: Sometimes]

Now, when you retire and try to sleep but cannot, try this--it works with me. You know when you are passing over your mental images become distorted and grotesque. I artificially induce that state. If I find myself rehearsing about two hundred times, with appropriate gestures, the keen, witty, logical remarks which I could have made in favor of my pet legislation in the club discussion, but didn't, then I begin after this fashion:

Pink elephants with green ribbons on their tails--red rhinoceri (is that right, or should it be rhinoceroses?)--smiling peanuts--Woman's City Club--Social Health Insurance--why didn't I say--I wish I had said--(here get out, you annoyance!)--pink elephants--and so forth and so forth.

[Sidenote: Picture of Pink Elephant Adorned]

[Sidenote: Woe Is Me]

Now I realize I have ruined myself. I am my own worst enemy. I have exposed my whole life before those modern vivisectionists, the army of amateur psycho-analysts.

[Sidenote: Exercise]

Third: Exercise. Great muscular exertion should be avoided, but the setting-up exercises that I advise, if begun with moderation and increased gradually, will undoubtedly stimulate the appetite and help the body functions to be better performed.

[Sidenote: Food]

Fourth: Since food is the only source of body substance, you must gradually train your stomach so that it can care for enough food to not only supply your bodily energy, but to leave a little excess to be stored as fat.

[Sidenote: Your Stomach]

If you have a small appetite--and many of you have--your stomach is undoubtedly contracted, and you must gradually add to the amount you have been eating, even though it may cause some distress, until you have disciplined it so that it can handle what you need without distress. The stomach is a muscular organ and can be trained and exercised somewhat as other organs can. You will not have much appetite at first, but it will develop. Sometimes a short fast for a day or two, drinking nothing but pure water, seems to be beneficial in the beginning.

Do not drink much with your meals, unless the drink has food value by the addition of lots of cream or sugar, or both.

[Sidenote: Eat More]

Decide how many calories you need for your activities, gradually add to your dietary until you have reached that number, and then some more, and you will gain as surely as the overweight individual will lose by doing the opposite. It may take a long time, or you may get results very rapidly, depending somewhat upon the individual characteristics. Gradually increase your butter, cream, sugar, chocolate, and so forth, as they are very high in food value.

Study the Key to the Calories and reckon your calories every day for a while. You have already noticed that the foods that you like are low in food value.

Here are some of the things you can take to add to your fuel:

[Sidenote: Try Some of These]

A glass of milk, hot or cold, taken between meals and before retiring, will add about 500 calories.

Cream sauce on your vegetables will add to their value.

Cod liver oil, or olive oil, or cream, begun in small doses and gradually increased.

One malted milk, made with milk, syrup, egg, ice cream, whipped cream, and the malted milk, will add about 500 calories.

[Sidenote: Learned Phraseology]

You remember the painful time that I spoke of when there was so much more of me than there ought to be? Well, the aforesaid concoction, made with milk, syrup, egg, ice cream, whipped cream, and the malted milk, was accessory before the fact, and also particeps criminis before the law.

I absorbed this phraseology by being president of the Professional Woman's Club, with its high-class women attorneys, ministers, dentists, Ph.D.'s, and "Medical Trust" doctors.

[Sidenote: Explanatory Note 1]

"Medical Trust."--The American Medical Association (A.M.A.), a powerful trust you can't get into unless you have a high preliminary education and are a graduate of a high-class medical college. Eleven years' training after the grammar school is their minimum standard now.

[Sidenote: Explanatory Note 2]

"League for Medical Ignorance."--The so-called "League for Medical Freedom"; the opponent of the above mentioned trust. Their standard--any old kind of a medical or religious training, two weeks or longer, engrafted on anyone who has the money to pay for the course. No education, no barrier; in fact, those of limited education make the loudest boosters for the league. In justice, I must say that many splendid, estimable persons belong to this league, not knowing these facts.

[Sidenote: Thorough Mastication]

Fifth: See page 92 in my advice to the fat. It is as important for you as for them. (It always makes me mildly furious when I look up a word and am directed to seek some other locality. If it affects you that way--seek page 60 in my advice to you.)

Also have your teeth X-rayed. Blind abscesses at the roots will cause all sorts of aches and pains, as well as underweight.

[Sidenote: Especially About Your Ailments]

[Sidenote: Organ Recitals Wednesday Evenings Only]

Sixth: Don't talk so much. See if you can't leave out two-thirds of the totally unimportant, uninteresting details. A tremendous amount of energy is used in talking. This habit I would not say was confined to you, by any means; it is another one of those pretty nearly universal errors.

I will not give you a sample fattening menu, for it might be all out of proportion to what you could handle, and it would upset you. Make out your own menus, realizing that you must work gradually to the desired amount.

I am taking it for granted that you are organically sound, that your scientific, educated physician has said there is nothing the matter with you, except perhaps your "nervous" disposition.

Have I not been nice to you? All right, relax and watch yourself get into the class of the plumptically adequate.

And if you don't succeed after a faithful trial, take the milk-cure, with its three to six weeks' absolute rest.

Recapitulation

1. Calm yourself. 2. Sleep. 3. Exercise. 4. Food. 5. Masticate 6. Delete the details. 7. Milk-cure.

Review

1. Repeat Elbert Hubbard's advice. 2. Give three reasons why worry can make you thin. 3. Define "Medical Trust" and "League for Medical Freedom." 4. Memorize paragraph about nature 5. Enumerate the things you can eat to increase your calories.

7

Exercise

It is practically impossible to reduce weight through exercise alone, unless one can do a tremendous amount of it. For the food that one eats is usually enough to cover the energy lost by the exercise.

[Sidenote: Light On Your Feet]

However, exercise is a very important feature of any reducing program; not because of the fat that is burned up in the exercise--and there is some burned--but for the reason that it is necessary to keep one in a healthy condition. The muscles, the internal organs, the bones, the brain, are all benefited--in fact, the entire system.

[Sidenote: Duty Dances]

The exercises described hereinafter will help make you fat or thin, and they will keep you supple, graceful, and light on your feet, so that when I tell my husband that he must dance with you, Madam, he will not say, "Nothing stirring," and when you, Professor, ask me to dance, I will not curse the day I was born.

[Sidenote: Warning]

If you have not been accustomed to exercise, I warn you to take up only one or two at a time and do each one a few times only. You will be atrociously sore, and you will realize that you have muscles of which you wotted not.

However, persist, if you are sure there are no organic reasons why you shouldn't--such as a weak heart. (In case you are very much overweight, I think it advisable to wait until you have reduced somewhat.)

[Sidenote: Or Classic Dancing]

It is splendid if you can belong to a gymnasium or to a physical culture class, but ten to fifteen minutes' systematic daily exercise practiced with vim, and each set followed by deep breathing, will do more good than a gymnasium spasmodically attended. Brisk walking with a long stride isn't so bad; in fact, if taken with a very long stride it will twist 'most every organ you have in your body.

There are hundreds of exercises you can take. If you will notice little rascal's illustrations you will find many good ones. Those illustrating the beginning of this chapter are excellent.

If possible, it is best to take the exercises on arising in the morning, but if you have a household to care for you may not be able to do so. For those who have to do their own work, it may be well to do the work first. You can do it in half the time if you plan it carefully and speed up. (This advice is not for my thin friends; their speedometers register too high already.) It does not matter so much when the exercises are done as that they are done, and done every day for the rest of your life, with the possible exception of two or three days a month.

Gallstones, permanent stiff joints, and other little things like that will have a hard time forming.

My Exercises

[Sidenote: They Reach Most of My Muscles]

(The services of my noted artist I was able to obtain with great difficulty, as he was engaged in the more important work of making a swagger stick. I finally secured him by the promise of an ice cream cone and twenty-three cents to go with his two cents so that he could buy a Thrift Stamp. He is given due credit on the title page.)

[Sidenote: Turn On Your Music]

These exercises executed with vim, vigor, and vip--deep breathing between each set--will take ten to fifteen minutes. Re-read my warning.

[Sidenote: Little Movements with Meanings All Their Own]

1. Feet together, arms outstretched, palms up, describe as large a circle as possible. Fine for round shoulders and fat backs. Do slowly and stretch fifteen times. Smile.

2. Arms outstretched, swing to right and to left as far as possible at least 15 times each.

[Sidenote: Important! Keep Facial Expression Throughout as per Artist's Idea]

3. Bend sideways, to right and left, alternately, as far as possible at least 15 times each.

4. Revolve the body upon the hips from right to left at least 10 times, and left to right the same.

5. Bend and touch the floor with your fingers, without bending your knees, at least 15 times.

6. Knee-bending exercise, at least 15 times. This is hard at first.

7. Hand on door or wall, swing each leg back and forth at least 15 times. To the side 15 times. Turn head, raise arm, and tense both.

[Sidenote: You Will Soon Be as Graceful as Annette]

8. Step on chair with each foot at least 10 times. This is good for calf and thigh muscles. After a while you won't look as though you needed a derrick to get onto a street car.

9. Arms on sides of chair. Come down and touch abdomen. Fine for back and abdomen. Fifteen times.

[Sidenote: It Has Been Called to My Attention that Bone Back Brushes Should Not Be Used by Some; i.e., There Is Danger in Affinities]

10. Brush hair vigorously at least 200 double strokes all over the head, N.S.E.W., using a brush in each hand.

[Sidenote: Good Exercise]

(Military brushes are best. If you can't purloin a set of your husband's, two ordinary brushes will do.) Now shake out the loose dandruff. This is one of the best exercises and must not be omitted, for it accomplishes two purposes. It is a good arm and chest exercise, and it gives a healthy scalp absolutely free from the dammdruff.

NOW

This for a few minutes, followed by this, the hot preferably at night.

8

At Last! How to Reduce

The title of this chapter indicates to whom it is addressed. All others please refrain from reading, for it is strictly private and confidential, and is intended only for those who need it.

You thin and you normal had better save it, though, for you may qualify later. You are keeping right on reading now! I'm surprised. I wanted to tell my fat friends that the first thing they have to do is to get control of their will power, and now I can't do it.

Somehow, will power with a layer of fat on it gets feeble. Don't laugh, you too thin! It gets worse than feeble, if there is no fat at all and the nervous system is starved, it--well, I won't say what it does, for I don't want to worry you.

[Sidenote: Now That Order Is Restored I Will Resume]

Will power, being feeble to a greater or less degree, must be bolstered and aided a bit, to begin with, so--

First Order

[Sidenote: Watch Your Weight!]

[Sidenote: Nature Always Counts]

Tell loudly and frequently to all your friends that you realize that it is unpatriotic to be fat while many thousands are starving, that you are going to reduce to normal, and will be there in the allotted time. If you belong to a club, round up the overweights and form a section. Call it the "Watch Your Weight--Anti-Kaiser Class." Tax the members sufficiently to buy a good, accurate pair of scales. Meet once a week to weigh. Wear approximately the same weight clothes, and weigh at the same time in relation to eating. Do this whether or not you belong to a club. Once or twice a week is often enough to weigh. Scales vary, so try to use the same ones.

Don't be discouraged if some day after you have dieted well you seem to have gained. Nature sometimes seems fiendish that way. The excess weight is probably due to a retention of water, and will not be permanent. However, don't depend upon this too often! Usually, if you have gained when you think you ought not to, it is because Nature has been counting calories and you haven't.

Have the members listed on a weight chart conspicuously placed near the scales, and record accurately the weight weekly.

```
+-------------------------------------------------+  | WATCH YOUR WEIGHT ANTI-KAISER  CLASS  |  +-------------------------------------------------+  |  |Normal| Weight on |  +------------------+------+----------------------------+  | Members' Names |Weight|Date|Date|Date|Date|Date|Date|  +------------------+------+----+----+---
```

```
-+----+----+----+ | | | | | | | | | +-----------------+------+----+----+----+----+----+----+
| | | | | | | | | +-----------------+------+----+----+----+----+----+----+ | | | | | | | | |
+-----------------+------+----+----+----+----+----+----+ | | | | | | | | | +----------------
+------+----+----+----+----+----+----+ | | | | | | | | | +-----------------+------+----+----
+----+----+----+----+
```

[Sidenote: No Funds for the Red Cross]

Those not reducing at least one pound per week to be fined soundly and the proceeds given to the Red Cross. That won't be a good way to raise funds for the chapter, though, for there will be no fines after the first week or so, when the members find what their maintenance diet should be and are consuming less than that.

I will explain this maintenance diet business. You shameless thin ones, call back your more polite comrades--this is important for all of you. (I shall also tell you more fully about this in the last chapter.)

[Sidenote: Maintenance Diet]

The maintenance diet is one which maintains you at your present weight, i.e., you are not gaining or losing. You may be over or under normal, but are staying there. The intake equals the outgo.

When you eat less than your maintenance diet, you are going to supply the deficiency with your own fat.

So commit yourself on your honor that you are going to reduce or perish--no joke; you can't tell how near you are to it if you are much overweight. There are two general stages of fatty heart. In the first stage the heart is surrounded by a blanket of fat, and it also penetrates between the muscles. Later, if it goes on too long, the heart muscle itself degenerates to fat, then--

[Sidenote: Good-night!]

Shakespeare warns you to make thy body less, hence thy grace more; leave gormandizing, and know that the grave doth gape for thee thrice wider than for other men.

Second Order

[Sidenote: Shrink Your Stomach]

Your stomach, long used to an excess of food for your needs--it may not be a large amount--but still, I repeat, being used to an excess of food for your needs, your stomach must be disciplined. It is undoubtedly distended, as it should not be.

[Sidenote: Shrink Your Stomach]

A good way to show it that you are master is to fast for at least one day-- drink nothing but pure water, hot or cold, as you prefer. It will protest vociferously and will tell all its friends, the different organs of your body, how you are persecuting it, and they will join the league against you and decide they will oust you from your position, and you will feel like--but don't mind it; it will soon know that you mean business, and, much chastened and considerably contracted, will take the next day a very small amount of food very gratefully.

[Sidenote: Shrink Your Stomach]

If you do not want to be so severe with it you can allow it five glasses of hot or cold skim milk or buttermilk, one every three hours, say, at 10,1,4,7, and 10 o'clock. One glass is 80 calories, five equal 400 calories, which is not so much.

[Sidenote: Or Mashed]

The baked potato and glass of skim milk diet, three times a day one day a week, which has its devotees, depends upon its low caloric content for its results. There is no magic in it, no yeast business which reduces. This is most wholesome, however, for potatoes contain a large amount of the potassium salts, which tend to counteract the effects of uric acid, and thus are good for the gouty type.

[Sidenote: Mono-Diets]

The beefsteak, the milk, and the fruit diets are also good. One can gain as well as lose on the milk diet, all depending on number of calories consumed, and it is an excellent method for both. The beefsteak diet is beneficial for a short time, but too much protein over a long period has been shown to be harmful. An exclusive fruit diet is excellent for reduction.

Low calorie days can be repeated once a week if necessary in order to keep the stomach in good order. Fruit juice, one-quarter glass, or fresh fruit, can be substituted for the skim milk, and you may prefer it.

[Sidenote: But You Do Not Have To]

You could keep on this for some time, or fast for some time, and probably be much benefited. I fasted five days once, or rather fruit-juiced five days. I lost about ten pounds, I think, and my heart, which had begun to carry on, was relieved.

[Sidenote: Sob Stuff]

It was during that period of which I have spoken, and of which I am ashamed; for I had my M.D. degree then and should have known better. But you know we have good authority that it is easier to teach twenty what were good to be done than to be one of twenty to follow our own teaching.

Third Order

[Sidenote: You Are Down to Business]

[Sidenote: And Maybe Diabetes]

Now you will have to reckon on the amount of food or number of calories you need per day. Review the rule I have given. You find for your age and normal weight that you will need, let us say for example, 2200 calories. You have probably been consuming twice that amount and either storing it away as fat or as disease. (It is surprising how small an excess will gradually add up pounds of fat. For instance, three pats of butter or three medium chocolate creams a day, if over the maintenance limit, would add approximately 27 pounds a year to your weight!)

Now you are to reduce your maintenance diet--the 2200 calories we are taking for example--to 1200 calories--quite a comfortable lot, you will find.

You will be surprised how much 1200 calories will be if the food is judiciously selected.

[Sidenote: After All, Hunger Is Much More Agreeable Than Apoplexy]

You may be hungry at first, but you will soon become accustomed to the change. I find that dry lemon or orange peel, or those little aromatic breath sweeteners, just a tiny bit, seem to stop the hunger pangs; or you may have a cup of fat-free bouillon or half an apple, or other low calorie food. (Count the calories here.)

One thousand calories less food per day equals four ounces of fat lost daily-- approximately 8 pounds per month. If you do not want to lose so fast, do not cut down so much.

Fourth Order

[Sidenote: You Register Joy]

You may eat just what you like--candy, pie, cake, fat meat, butter, cream--but--count your calories! You can't have many nor large helpings, you see; but isn't it comforting to know that you can eat these things? Maybe some meal you would rather have a 350-calorie piece of luscious pie, with a delicious 150-calorie tablespoonful of whipped cream on it, than all the succulent vegetables Luther Burbank could grow in California.

My idea of heaven is a place with me and mine on a cloud of whipped cream.

[Sidenote: You Registered Too High]

Now that you know you can have the things you like, proceed to make your menus containing very little of them.

Fifth Order

This is going to be your chief business and pursuit in life for the next few months, this reducing of your weight. However, keep up your Red Cross and all other activities, fast and furiously, so that you won't be thinking about yourself.

[Sidenote: More Warnings]

Don't reduce more than two or three pounds a week; two or less is better. If you are too cannibalistic, your heart, kidneys and nervous system are liable to suffer--you yourself are supplying too much fat in your dietary, and there are other scientific reasons against reducing too rapidly.

However, you may find that the first week or so you may reduce five or seven pounds; but don't worry about this, for that is a slushy, watery fat that goes easily.

If a claim like a cold should attack you, and after spraying nose and throat frequently with an antiseptic, and then denying the claim vigorously, it persists in running a severe course, better go back to maintenance diet for a few days.

[Sidenote: Not Even While Cooking]

Don't "taste"! You will find the second taste much harder to resist than the first. If you have allowed in your daily program something between meals (a good plan), take it, but not otherwise.

Try not to overeat at any time, and thus undo the work that perhaps has taken you two or three days to accomplish. It will be all right occasionally, possibly one day a week, to eat up to your maintenance diet, but don't, I beg of you, go over it so that you will gain.

You will be tempted quite frequently, and you will have to choose whether you will enjoy yourself hugely in the twenty minutes or so that you will be consuming the excess calories, or whether you will dislike yourself cordially for the two or three days you lose by your lack of will power.

[Sidenote: I Ought Not to Do This]

I am afraid I am going to tell a story. I feel as though I were, and I don't want to. It is one I heard years ago at a teachers' convention at Riverside, when I was a tender, unsuspecting young school teacher, so it is perfectly good, albeit senile--and it illustrates my point so well--so well--well, you have to put yourself in the place of the little chaps, Billie and Johnnie, of the kindergarten.

[Sidenote: A Little Anatomical Story]

It seems it was customary to bring a lunch, and Little-new-boy had come without one. Teacher asked Billie would he share? No, sturdily; not he. But little Johnnie, he would. Some time later, Johnnie, with a frantic waving of his hand, and with just pride in his generosity, informed the class that he had shared his lunch with Little-new-boy and he felt good is his little heart.

Billie stood his ground and stoutly declared that he ate his and he felt good in his little belly.

9

Autobiographical

I did not give our thin friends a sample menu for fear it would upset them; but nothing can upset your digestion, I know. However, I will not give you a sample menu, either, but will tell you what I eat when I go on a reduction regime, which for me is 1200 Calories.

You will notice, most of my calories I have at dinner in the evening. You may not like this, but would rather have yours spread over the entire day; and you can suit your fancy, for it makes no difference as long as your total number per day stays within your reduction limit.

[Sidenote: Make Out Several Menus if You Like]

Don't think you have to follow my menu. You might gain on it! Study the Key and select your own.

Many will lose by going on the no-breakfast plan, or the no-lunch plan. If they do reduce, it is because they have lowered their daily consumption of food, and not because of the no-breakfast or no-lunch plan per se.

Fat seems to melt faster when the chief meal is in the middle of the day, and with only 200 or 300 calories of fruit for the evening meal. In this way you slim while you sleep.

MY BREAKFAST

1 slice very dry coarse bread toast 1/4 in. thick 50 C. Butter, 1/4 cu. in 25 C. Hot water flavored with coffee 00 C. ----- Total 75 C.

[Sidenote: Slim While You Sleep! Clever?]

You may prefer many more calories for breakfast, or none at all. This may not look good to you, but it means an awful lot in my young life, after my exercise and bath, to sit down to my little breakfast and read the papers.

Recently I have found that two cups of moderately hot water with the juice of a lemon answers just as well as the toast and watery coffee, and is probably better. You might like some fruit.

MY LUNCHEON

1 corn muffin--I am patriotic 125 C. 1 pat butter 100 C. 1 cup coffee with 1 tbsp. cream 50 C. ------ Total 275 C.

If you are patriotic and constipated, substitute one bran muffin. You can see that this is in reality a further extension of my sumptuous breakfast. If I get tired of this, I add a salad of

Lettuce, large amount, practically 00 C. Roquefort cheese dressing 100 C.

I am very fond of this Roquefort cheese dressing; 1-1/8in. cube of cheese in a little vinegar, no oil, keeps it within the hundred calories.

You might prefer a baked apple or two tomatoes, or a dish of prunes, or 3 oz. of cottage cheese. The chief thing is to take what you like, not what I like. Count your calories.

MY DINNER

[Sidenote: I Don't Mean Your Husband's Dessert, I Mean My Husband's. My Word! I Got Out of That Quick!]

Vegetable soup, or bouillon, no fat; or small oyster cocktail 25 C. Lean meat, or "unthinking" lobster or fish, 5 or 6 oz 300 C. Large serving of uncooked lettuce or cabbage, practically 00 C. Mayonnaise or oil, 1/2 dsp 50 C. 1 large dish tomatoes, or cauliflower, or string beans, or carrots, or turnips (I hate turnips--just put them down so you can see you can have them if you like) 25 C. 1 medium slice bread, or 1 medium potato 100 C. 1 pat butter 100 C. 100 calories of your husband's dessert 100 C. Water 00 C. 1 cup cereal coffee, clear, practically 00 C. -------- Total 700 C.

SUMMARY

Breakfast 75 C. Luncheon including salad 375 C. Dinner 700 C. ------- 1150 C.

That leaves me 50 more calories to total 1200, to take before retiring if I am hungry. You should leave this 50 calories to take before retiring, because if you are hungry you will find it very difficult to go to sleep.

A small cup of hot skimmed milk tends to be a sedative. Hunger, like cold feet, is hard to go to sleep on.

[Sidenote: For Both Sexes]

If there is one thing more important than another, it is thorough mastication.

[Sidenote: Sometimes I Take More Than 100 Calories of My Husband's Dessert. I Love Fat Men, But I Don't Want to Be Married to 'Em]

This applies to the thin as well as to the fat, and to the child as well as to the adult. Take a moderate mouthful and rassel with it until it is automatically swallowed. Chew until it is all gone before you put any more in your mouth. There is no better way of jollying yourself into thinking that you have had all you want than this Fletcherizing habit, and it takes the same time to consume one-half the amount of food you have been in the habit of eating.

I will allow you all the water you want, in reason; in fact, I advise it while you are reducing, both at the meals and between meals. The only precaution is that at the meals it should not be drunk while food is in the mouth, for this would tend to lessen thorough mastication.

Now, Madam and Madam's husband, when are you going to begin this important business of reducing? After the holidays? Tomorrow? No! Right now. The sooner you get started, the better. The chief thing to do, and the hardest, is to get started and to get the habit. After the first three days you will not dread it; in fact; you will feel so much better that you will not be willing to go back to your old habits of overeating.

Now let's review a bit what you are to do.

[Sidenote: Plan the Day Before]

First: Pledge yourself to yourself, and to someone else, so you will be ashamed to fail. There is a great deal of psychology to reducing. Use strong auto-suggestion. Decide just how much you are going to eat in advance of the meal--so many calories, no more! This sounds foolish, but it helps wonderfully.

Second: Begin with a fast or a low caloric diet for the first day; keep it, if necessary, one day weekly.

[Sidenote: Low Bridge on Fats and Pastries]

Third: Study food list and make out menus the caloric totals of which are less than your maintenance diet. Have a fairly balanced diet, some fat, some carbohydrates, some protein, and a good amount of green vegetables and fruit. Have 200-300 C's of protein.

Fourth: Masticate every morsel with such thoroughness that it is automatically swallowed.

Fifth: Keep up your activities--Red Cross and other relief work.

Sixth: Remember that you will feel good in your little heart when you resist temptation to overeat, and when you don't, you won't feel good anywhere.

Seventh: Some vigorous exercise every day.

[Sidenote: There Is Life Substance and Intelligence in Chocolate Creams!]

NOTE: If there comes a time when you think you will die unless you have some chocolate creams, go on a c.c. debauch. I do, occasionally, and will eat as many as ten or so; but I take them before dinner, then me for the balance of my dinner--

1 bowl of clear soup 25 C. 1 cracker 25 C. ------ Total 50 C.

And thus, you see, every supposed pleasure in sin (eating) will furnish more than its equivalent of pain (dieting) until belief in material life (chocolate creams) is destroyed.

Review

1. Describe your stomach.

2. If there is one thing more important than another, what is it?

3. Repeat the five orders in chapter 8.

4. Repeat the warnings.

5. Work the following example:

X gains 25 pounds during the year. How many calories has he averaged daily over his maintenance diet?

KEY:

25 lbs. fat = 400 oz. fat. 1 oz. fat represents 275 C. food consumed. 400 oz. = 400 x 275, or 110,000 C. 110,000 ?365 = 301 C. Answer. X has eaten 301 C. per day more than necessary.

6. How many calories have you averaged daily over your maintenance diet? And what could you have left off your menu and kept from gaining all that weight?

10

Testimonials

[Sidenote: From the Field]

After you have reduced or gained, let me share your joys. Write me a little note. You need not sign your name if you don't want to. I anticipate the following:

DEAR DOCTOR:

I am so grateful to you, Dr. Lulu Hunt Peters, for what you have done for me. After reading your book, "Diet and Health, with Key to the Calories" my chronic case of meanness--I mean leanness--was absolutely cured. My weight, which was ... now is ... and I am on my way to normal. I am fond of you.

* * * * *

DEAREST DOCTOR:

I cannot be too grateful to you, dear Doctor Lulu Hunt Peters, for your book "Diet and Health, with Key to the Calories," for I have lost ... pounds! My weight was ... and now is ... and I am on my way to normal.

I should be ungrateful indeed if I did not mention that while reading the book a chronic case of dammdruff which I had had for years, and which had been given up by six specialists, was absolutely cured. I adore you!

* * * * *

[Sidenote: A Wonderful Demonstration]

DEAR DOCTOR:

For your book, "Diet and Health, with Key to the Calories," words are inadequate to express my thanks. For I have been delivered from a chronic affliction of many years' duration, for which I had tried all known methods of cure. I refer to the smoking of cheap cigars by my husband. He suddenly found he had no desire for the noxious weed! Your arm and leg exercises are wonderful.

* * * * *

11

An Apology and Some Amendments

On re-reading this literary gem, humorous classic, and scientific treatise on weight reduction and gaining, I see that I have a very intimate mixture of the thins and the fats. But that is as it should be for balance. I had intended to keep you strictly separate, but the preaching, the exercises, the dry definitions, the Key to the Calories, and so forth, was matter that was applicable to both, so it could not be done.

[Sidenote: Watch Your Weight]

I have just got to bring this to a close now, if I have it ready as I promised, for the lecture, "Watch Your Weight!" I am glad of it, too. I am getting so ... funny it is painful. I will close with the next chapter. It will be beautifully scientific, but not funny, I promise.

Some Amendments

[Sidenote: No. 1]

You perhaps have noticed that my first chapter is called "Preliminary Bout," and then I have gone on to describe a club meeting. I am aware that P.B. is a prize fighting term, and I meant it for the picture of me fighting myself, not for the club meeting. I have attended many club meetings, and in none of them have I ever seen any fighting that would have taken any prize anywhere, although I will say I have seen and have myself personally conducted some very classy stuff.

[Sidenote: No. 2]

I do not use slang. I use only the purest, most refined, and cultured English. I leave slang to those who can get by with it and put it over. So where I have used dashes you may use your favorite slang words. Mine were deleted by the censors.

[Sidenote: No. 3 (a)]

Mrs. Ima Gobbler is not really fat enough to be called a fat--! She is only 40 or 50 pounds overweight, but she is fond of me and I took liberties with her. She is a darling.

[Sidenote: No. 3 (b)]

She is a purist, too. I called her up after I put her in my book, and I said, "You are fond of me, aren't you, Mrs. Gobbler?" And she said, "Youbetcha." "And you are a good sport, aren't you?" "Surest thing you know!" "That's good, for I have said a horrid thing to you. I had to, in order to stop the club discussion." And she responded soulfully, "Go to it, Kid!"

[Sidenote: No. 4]

Mrs. Sheesasite's husband did not really have to buy her a pair of freight scales; that is just a gentle josh. The ordinary scales will weigh 300 pounds, I believe. She is also a dear.

[Sidenote: No. 5]

My husband's eyes are not really green, nor is he cross-eyed. They are the loveliest, softest brown. The green eyes belong on the maternal side of this house.

[Sidenote: No. 6]

My artist is not really noted. He is just an ordinary adorable ten-year-old boy kiddie. Aren't his little figures the dearest ever?

* * * * *

[Sidenote: Doing My Bit]

All the characters in my book are friends of mine. Perhaps you had better substitute were for are. There was one woman mentioned in my original manuscript and my husband said what have you put her in for Pattie? (a corruption of Pettie, a H.moon hangover) she is no friend of yours: she knocks you. And I said loftily like, I want you to know Ijit (corruption of Idiot, also a H.moon hangover) I am above personalities she is prominent and besides she is fat especially in the feet and head and she doesn't know it and he said that doesn't make any difference you do not have to immortalize her and I said I would look up the authorities on the subject and he said he was authority enough and I said I would see what the other authorities said anyway and I did and I found one most eminent that said you should love your enemies but none that said you should immortalize them so I said I'd drop her and he said he should say so and so I did.

[Illustration: Dear Enemy Unimmortalised]

--All the characters in my book are friends of mine. Perhaps you had better substitute were for are.

12

Maintenance Diet and Conclusions

[Illustration: Maintenance Diet 1000 C. over 1000 C. under]

[Sidenote: 1st Circle]

THE HEAVY circle represents the amount of daily food (number of calories) which will maintain you at present weight. It may be your weight is too much or too little, but this is your maintenance diet for that weight.

[Sidenote: 2nd Circle]

THE SECOND circle represents a daily diet containing more than necessary for maintenance; for example, let us say 1000 calories more. This 1000 calories of food is equivalent to approximately 4 ounces of fat [1000?55 (1 oz. fat = 255 C.)]; 4 ounces of fat daily equals 8 pounds a month which will be added to your weight, and, if not needed by the system, will deposit itself as excess fat.

Or the toxins arising from the unnecessary food will irritate the blood vessels, causing arterio-sclerosis (hardening of the arteries), which in turn may cause kidney disease, heart disease, or apoplexy (rupture of artery in the brain), and maybe death before your time.

On the other hand, if you are underweight and the added nourishment is gradually worked up to, it will improve the health and cause a gain of so much (theoretically, and in reality if kept up long enough).

[Sidenote: 3d Circle]

THE THIRD circle represents a diet containing less than the maintenance; again, for example, say 1000 calories less. Here the 1000 calories must be taken from the body tissue, and fat is the first to go, for fat is virtually dead tissue.

This 4 ounces of fat daily which will be supplied by your body equals in six months 48 pounds.

There are in America hundreds of thousands of overweight individuals; not all so much overweight as this, but some considerably more so. If these individuals will save 1000 calories of food daily by using their stored fat, think what it would mean at this time.

[Sidenote: Savings]

Not only an immense saving of food to be sent to our soldiers and allies and the starving civilians, and of money which could be used for Liberty Bonds, the Red Cross, and other war relief work, but a great saving and a great increase in power; for there is no doubt that by reducing as slowly and scientifically as I have directed, efficiency and health will be increased one hundred fold.

If, as illustrated in the third circle, the 1000 calories or less is eaten and the individual already is underweight, with no excess fat, then this amount will be taken from the muscles and the more vital tissues, and the organism will finally succumb. Before this time is reached there will be a great lowering of resistance, and the individual will be a prey to the infectious diseases.

It must be remembered that in children the growth of the whole body is tremendously active, and especially that of the heart and nervous system.

If the nervous system is undernourished, it becomes disorganized and undeveloped. This is apt to be expressed in uncertain emotional states, quick tempers, and a predisposition to convulsions. The heart, if undernourished, lays its foundation for future heart disease, and the whole system will be injured for life.

Anything that impairs the vigor and vitality of children strikes at the basis of national welfare.

[Sidenote: The Food Administration Emphasizes This]

You can see from this how extremely important it is that, in our need for the conservation of food, only those who can deny themselves and at the same time improve their health and efficiently should do it. It will be no help in our crisis if the health and resistance of our people be lowered and the growth and development of our children be stunted.

We, the hundreds of thousands of overweight citizens, combined with the hundreds of thousands of the normal who are overeating to their ill, can save all the food that is necessary. We are anxious, willing, eager to do this. Now we know how, and we will.

Food Will Win the War

WATCH OUR WEIGHT!

13

Three Years Later

February, 1, 1921

An Added Chapter in Which Are Offered Twenty-one Suggestive Menus

After nearly two years with the American Red Cross in the Balkans I return to find the little book has been carrying on in my absence--I write this for the fifth edition--and my publishers insisting that I must furnish some more menus. They affirm that there are many who do not care to or cannot figure out their own.

After being so long under military discipline I obey now instinctively, although I do not want to do this. But you know publishers. They say that if there are menus for those who do not have the desire to compute them, the usefulness of the book will be increased. Publishers are so altruistic.

Now far be it from me to scorn the possibility of increased sales myself. So I comply, and after you are reduced you will have the energy and the increased keenness to scout around in the calories and make out your own.

* * * * *

A little of my Balkan experience in the reducing line may not be amiss. In Albania, where I was stationed most of the time, life is very strenuous. We all had to work hard and expend a great deal of nervous energy. Medical calls on foot in the scorching sun over unkind cobblestones, long distance calls on unkinder mules, long hours in nerve-racking clinics, ferocious man-eating mosquitos, scorpions, centipedes, sandflies, and fleas, and other unspeakable animals kept us hopping and slapping and scratching.

But there was one consolation to me. With this work, more intensive and more strenuous than I had ever done before, I would not have to diet--I would not have to watch my weight--I would not have to count my calories! Oh, joy!

We lived a community life, we Red Crossers. We had plain blunt food, American canned mostly, supplemented with the fare that could be eked out of Albania, and cooked by an Albanese who could not be taught that we Americans were not Esquimos and did not like food swimming in fat. However, it tasted good to famished Red Crossers, and I ate three meals a day, confident that I would retain my girlish middle-aged slenderness and not have to diet. We had no scales and no mirrors larger than our hand mirrors. Our uniforms were big and comfortable.

* * * * *

The French who are in charge of Scutari depart, the officers leaving to us some of their furniture, including a full length French plate mirror. Ordinarily when I look in a full-length mirror I don't hate myself so much--so it is with some degree of anticipated pleasure that I complacently approach, to get a life-size reflection of myself after many months of deprivation of that pleasure.

"Mon Dieu!" I exclaim. "Bogomi!" (Serbian--'For the love of Allah!') "This is no mirror," I mutter. "This is one of those musee things that make you look like a Tony Sarg picture of Irvin Cobb."

"What's irritating you, Dockie?" asks one of the girls, coming up and standing back of me. I look at her reflection. She does not look like Irvin Cobb!

"Peggy," I say tragically, "Peggy, do I look like my reflection?"

"Yes, dear, we have all noticed how stout you have been getting. Aren't you supposed to be some shark on the subject of ideal weight?"

And the bitter truth is borne in upon me--no matter how hard I work--no matter how much I exercise, no matter what I suffer, I will always have to watch my weight, I will always have to count my calories.

This is what I did then:

I stopped going to the breakfast table. I kept some canned milk and coffee in my room, and made me two cups of coffee. For lunch I ate practically what I wanted, limiting myself to one slice of bread or one potato (we had no butter), with fruit for dessert. For dinner I came down only when the dessert was being served, and had a share of that with some coffee. I was jeered and derided. You know how in community life we all are as disagreeable as we like, and still love each other. Did not I know the desserts were the most fattening part of the meal? I was some authority on how to reduce, I was!

In vain I told them that it did not matter so long as my total caloric intake did not equal the number that I needed. It was not until some months after, when they saw that I was normal weight again, that they began to realize I knew whereof I spoke.

Then came our withdrawal from Albania and release from duty. After months of canned goods came Paris with its famous dishes; Crème d'Isigny avec crème! Artichauts an beurre! Patisseries francaises! Oo lala! Again I said calories be dashed! I can reduce when I get home. I had no delusions now, you see.

* * * * *

And now I am home trying to help raise the funds for the starving children of Central Europe, and explaining to my friends that while there is a food shortage in Europe it is not because I was there; and that I am reducing and the money that I can save will help keep a child from starving, and that they can do the same; that for every pang of hunger we feel we can have a double joy, that of knowing we are saving worse pangs in some little children, and that of knowing that for every pang we feel we lose a pound. A pang's a pound the world around we'll say.

Every once in a while you hear that the caloric theory has been exploded. There is no caloric "theory." Therefore none to explode. Calories are simply units for measuring heat and energy and never will be exploded any more than the yard or meter "theory" will be exploded. Foods must contain essential salts and the growth and health maintaining elements. These cannot be measured by calories. The quantity of heat or energy production but not the quality of the foods is measured in calories, and one must have a knowledge of the qualities also. No scientifically educated individual has ever thought otherwise.

The chief objection to following the advice of the numerous laymen who write eat-and-grow-thin menus is that they advise the elimination of all fats, sugars and starches. They lose sight of the fact, or they do not know, that the obese individual--I dislike that term--will have to have a balanced diet even while reducing if he is to maintain his health. One will lose weight on these menus, but as very many can testify they lose their health also. One cannot live on an unbalanced diet for any length of time without becoming unbalanced also. And furthermore the over-weighter will always have to diet more or less, and will have to have menus which he can continue to use. After normal weight is reached he will not have to be nearly so abstemious, but the same dietetic errors which produced overweight in the first place will produce it again. So he must know something of dietetics and he must have a balanced diet.

Now I shall make out some balanced menus, 1200 C's a day, being careful to include a large amount of the leafy vegetables and some milk or its products, the foods that McCollom calls PROTECTIVE FOODS because they contain in a large measure the essential mineral salts, and those vital elements he has called "Fat soluble A" and "Water soluble B"--others call vitamines--which he has proved to be so vital and necessary for growth in the young and the maintenance of health in the adult. I shall also include 200-300 C's of protein.

The leafy vegetables, cabbage, cauliflower, celery tops, lettuce, onion, Swiss chard, turnip tops, and other leaves employed as greens, water cress, etc., not only contain these vital elements, but they also exert a favourable influence on sluggish bowels and kidneys. They are low in caloric value, hence are low in fat-producing properties, and can be consumed with indiscretion, properly masticated.

It is better while you are reducing to stay away from the dining table when you do not expect to eat. If you are rooming, get a tiny sterno outfit, some substitute or coffee, some canned or dry milk, some sugar if you use it, and you can make a hot drink in your room and be independent for your breakfast and your evening meal, when you decide some day to go without that. Do not take more than 100 calories for your breakfast. That leaves you 1100 calories to be divided during the day if you go on a 1200 calorie schedule. I suggest the following distribution of the calories:

Breakfast 100 C's. Lunch 350 " Tea 100 " Dinner 650 "

You can reverse the dinner and lunch if you desire. If you do so then have your 100 calories I have allowed for tea time to take just before you retire. On a 1200 calorie schedule arranged as I have it you will not be hungry, I assure you. It will not be more than three or four days before your stomach will be shrunk and this amount I have allowed you will almost seem like overeating! That is the big idea. Shrink your stomach. Go on a fast or low calorie day for a day if necessary to get started. See page 81.

I can safely say that any up and around adult will reduce on 1200 calories, for that will not supply the basal metabolism, i.e., the body's internal activities, such as the beating of the heart, respiration, digestion, excretion, etc., and some of the body's stored fat will be called upon to supply the deficiency. How much one will reduce depends on how many calories are actually needed for the internal and the external activities. See pages 26 and 27. It is not advisable to reduce too rapidly. See page 85.

Now you have 1200 calories a day to eat. Let us think of this in terms of money. You have a limited amount of money every day to spend for food. You must spend it judiciously and get the food you need and want. If you spend the most of it on one article you have that much less for other things. It is possible that some days you will want to spend more than your allowance and you draw on your next day's supply. That will be all right if you remember that you have done so and will spend that much less the next day to equalize your account. You must study to spend wisely and carefully so as to supply your needs, but you cannot spend more than you have without restitution and retribution. Here are the menus:

BREAKFASTS

100 C. Each

1. Fruit 2 med. apples or 1 baked apple with 2 tsps. sugar or 1 large orange or 1/2 large grapefruit or 1 small cup berries or 1/2 good sized cantaloupe or 2 med. figs or 5 prunes

2. 1 cup coffee or cereal coffee.. O 1 tbsp. cream...................50 C 2 small tsp. sugar.............50 C or 2 cups with cream alone or sugar alone ---- Total..........................100 C

3. 10 ozs. skim milk hot or cold or 5 ozs. whole milk......................100 C

4. 1 cup coffee clear............. 0 1 thin slice toast.............75 C 1/4 pat butter.................25 C ---- Total............................100 C

Note--The skim milk breakfasts and teas are most desirable because of the protein content.

TEAS

100 C. Each See lists for breakfasts. Also could have:

1. 1 cup tea with 1 tsp. sugar 1 slice lemon.................25 C 3 soda crackers...............75 C ---- Total....................................100 C

2. 2 small plain cookies tea no cream or sugar................100 C

3. 1 chocolate cream 1 cup tea or hot water no cream or sugar....................100 C

* * * * *

The following combinations need not be followed arbitrarily. You may change them around if you desire. Look in the calorie lists for substitutes of the same classes of foods, if you do not like my combinations. If you don't care for the 100 C's at tea time you may have that much more for dinner.

1200 C DAY

ON ARISING

2 cups hot water with a little lemon juice. 10-minute exercise at least

BREAKFAST

Coffee or postum with cream or sugar or 10 ozs. skim milk (see list of breakfasts). 100 C

LUNCH

1 medium sized head lettuce 1/3 lb............................ 25 C 1 tbsp. mayonnaise................100 C 1 med. sweet pickle chopped for mayonnaise....................... 25 C 1-1/8 inch cube cream cheese melted or 3 ozs. cottage cheese............100 C 1 Toasted French roll (no butter) ....100 C -----

Total................................350 C

TEA

3 crackers with tea and 1 tsp. sugar and 1 slice lemon or 10 ozs. skim or buttermilk or 100 C. fruit (see list).................100 C

DINNER

Creamed dried beef on toast Dried beef 4 thin slices 4 x 5.100 C Cut fine and crisped in frying pan with 1/2 tbsp. butter.........50 C 1 tbsp. flour browned with above........................25 C Add 1 cup skim milk (7 ozs.) cook gently.....................70 C ----- 245 C

2 slices crisp toast (pour above over).........................200 C 1 large serving raw celery or raw cabbage.....................15 C 1 large baked apple with 1 tbsp. syrup.........................120 C 1 glass skim milk (7 oz.).........70 C

Total......................650 C ------- Grand Total................1200 C

1200 C DAY

ON ARISING

2 cups hot water, with a little lemon juice. 10-minute exercise at least

BREAKFAST Coffee or postum with cream or sugar or 10 ozs. skim milk (see list of breakfasts)...........................100 C

LUNCH

Celery--eat tender leaves also 10-14 stalks....................30 C Olives--5 good sized ripe.......100 C 1 small slice corn bread........100 C 12 ozs. skim milk or buttermilk.120 C ----- Total....................350 C

TEA

3 crackers with tea with 1 tsp. sugar and 1 slice lemon or 10 ozs. skim milk or buttermilk or 100 C fruit (see list)..................100 C

DINNER

Broiled halibut (or lean beef) steak 4-5 ozs. with lemon........150 C Lettuce (no oil) average serving....0 1 slice whole wheat bread or roll.100 C 1/2 pat butter......................50 C Dessert 1-6 pie....................350 C 1 cup clear postum or coffee........0 ----- Total....................650 C ------- Grand Total............1200 C

1200 C DAY

ON ARISING

2 cups hot water with a little lemon juice. 10-minute exercise at least

BREAKFAST

Coffee or postum with cream or sugar or 10 ozs. skim milk (see list of breakfasts) ....100 C

LUNCH

Combination salad Shredded lettuce 10 leaves......0 1 large tomato.................50 C 6 stalks chopped celery........15 C tender leaves included 1/2 med. cucumber..............15 C 1 med. grated carrot...........20 C ---- 100 C

1/2 tbsp. mayonnaise or oil......50 C with vinegar or lemon 1 slice whole wheat bread.......100 C 10 ozs. skim milk or buttermilk.100 C -----

Total.................................350 C

TEA

3 crackers with tea with 1 tsp. sugar and 1 slice lemon or 10 ozs. skim milk or buttermilk or 100 C fruit (see list).................100 C

DINNER

Croquettes of split peas or beans 1/2 cup mashed beans or peas 1/4 cup toast crumbs 1 tsp. cream or canned milk made into croquettes and baked or broiled.................225 C Stewed tomatoes 8 ozs. or 1 large fresh tomato.............50 C 1 slice bread or 5 small pretzels......................100 C 1 double serving lettuce or chopped cabbage or cauliflower.15 C 1 slice lemon, custard or squash pie, no top crust.............260 C 1 cup clear coffee or postum......0 -----

Total..........................650 C ----- Grand Total...................1200 C

1200 C DAY

ON ARISING

2 cups hot water with a little lemon juice. 10-minute exercise at least

BREAKFAST

Coffee or postum with cream or sugar or 10 ozs. skim milk (see list of breakfasts)...........................100 C

LUNCH

Fruit salad 1 large orange..................100 C 1 average apple.................50 C 1 small banana..................100 C 2 tbsps. lemon juice............10 C 2 small teasps. sugar...........40 C ----- 300 C Sprinkle with 1 tbsp. grapenuts..50 C

Total.........................350 C

TEA

3 crackers with tea with 1 tsp. sugar and 1 slice lemon or 10 ozs. skim milk or buttermilk or 100 C. fruit (see list)................100 C

DINNER

12 moderate sized oysters..............100 C Dipped in 1 beaten egg and crumbs of 3 crackers.........150 C Fried gently in 1 tbsp. of bacon or other fat...........125 C ----- 375 C 2 small slices crisped bacon.....50 C 1 small dish chow chow with lettuce.........................25 C 1 slice bread or its equivalent.100 C 1/2 pat butter..................50 C Dessert 1 medium baked apple with no sugar.................50 C ----- Total........................650 C ------ Grand Total.................1200 C

1200 C DAY

ON ARISING

2 cups hot water with a little lemon juice. 10-minute exercise at least

BREAKFAST

Coffee or postum with cream or sugar

or

10 ozs. skim milk (see list of breakfasts) ....100 C

LUNCH

2 eggs 160 C fried gently in 1 tsp. bacon fat or butter............40 C

or

soft boiled or poached eggs with 1 slice crisped bacon....200 C 1 roll or 1 slice whole wheat bread.........................100 C Butter 1/2 pat...................50 C Coffee, postum or tea clear.......0 ----- Total...................................350 C

TEA

3 crackers with tea with 1 tsp. sugar and 1 slice lemon

or

10 ozs. skim milk or buttermilk

or

100 C fruit (see list)..................100 C

DINNER

2 toasted shredded wheat biscuits.200 C 2 glasses skim milk...............150 C 1 dish stewed prunes 8 with 1 tbsp. syrup............200 C 10-12 peanuts.....................100 C Coffee, postum or tea clear.........0 C ----- Total...............................650 C ----- Grand Total..........................1200 C

1200 C DAY

ON ARISING

2 cups hot water with a little lemon juice. 10-minute exercise at least

BREAKFAST

Coffee or postum with cream or sugar

or

10 ozs. skim milk (see list of breakfasts) ....100 C

LUNCH

6 oz. cream soup, Potato, tomato, clam chowder, etc. (use skim milk)..........200 C Shredded cabbage, lettuce, celery

or

any greens--average helping practically....................0 C 1/2 tbsp. mayonnaise or oil

or

1 tbsp. cream dressing...........50 C 2 soda crackers..................50 C 1 average

apple..................50 C ----- Total..................................350 C

TEA

3 crackers with tea with 1 tsp. sugar and 1 slice lemon

or

10 ozs. skim milk or buttermilk

or

100 C fruit (see list)..................100 C

DINNER

Carrot and cottage cheese salad (The Home Dietitian--Comstock) 1/2 cup ground carrots 1-6 cup chopped nuts 3 oz. cottage cheese 3 oz. large lemon (juice of)......250 C 8 ozs. consomme, no fat...............30 C 4 crackers or 1 roll or slice bread 100 C 1/2 pat butter........................50 C Average helping lettuce or other greens--no oil......................0 Dessert--gelatine pudding, average serving...................120 C Whipped cream 1 heaping tbsp........100 C Coffee or postum or tea clear....... 0 ----- Total....................................650 C ------ Grand Total............................1200 C

1200 C DAY

ON ARISING

2 cups hot water with a little lemon juice. 10-minute exercise at least

BREAKFAST

Coffee or postum with cream or sugar or 10 ozs. skim milk (see list of breakfasts)........................100 C

LUNCH

Baked beans if canned 3 h. tbsp., if home baked 1-1/2........................150 C Pickled beets 5 med. slices......... 25 C Large amount celery or lettuce or other green leaves............. 25 C 1 slice toasted Swedish health bread (made of oatmeal) or 1 roll............................100 C 1 cup coffee or postum clear......... 0 C Medium apple........................ 50 C ----- Total............................350 C

TEA

3 crackers with tea with 1 tsp. sugar and 1 slice lemon or 10 ozs. skim milk or buttermilk or 100 C fruit (see list)....................100 C

DINNER

Cottage cheese omelet 2 med. eggs........................160 C 3 ozs. cottage cheese.............100 C 1 tbsp. cream or condensed milk..................... 50 C ----- 310 C

Salt to taste Bake or fry gently in 1/2 tbsp. fat. 40 C (Can substitute 100 C chopped lean meat for cottage cheese) 1 small head celery tender leaves and all............. 25 C 1 slice bread or equivalent......... 100 C Butter 1/2, pat..................... 50 C 1 dish plain stewed tomatoes, squash, carrots, spinach or onions, etc....................... 25 C 5 almonds or 5 peanuts or 2 large walnuts..................... 50 C 10 raisins......................... 50 C ----- Total............................650 C ------ Grand Total.....................1200 C

Finished But Not Famished

Printed in the USA
CPSIA information can be obtained
at www.ICGtesting.com
CBHW051706211024
16187CB00039B/1539